Forget Alzheimer's

Forget Alzheimer's

WHAT'S BEHIND US PATENT 8,708,906 B1, "METHOD FOR THE PREVENTION OF DEMENTIA AND ALZHEIMER'S DISEASE"

Allen J Orehek M.D.

ISBN-13: 9781506191539
ISBN-10: 1506191533
Library of Congress Control Number: 2015905359
CreateSpace Independent Publishing Platform
North Charleston, South Carolina

Contents

Introduction

"Simply because a medical problem is very
common does not make it normal."
—ALLEN J. OREHEK, MD

This book is designed to be your tool for the prevention of dementia. In 2014, the United States Patent Office issued "Method for the Prevention of Dementia and Alzheimer's Disease" (patent number US 8,708,906 B1) to Allen J. Orehek, MD.

As a physician of medicine, I enthusiastically dedicate myself to understanding and developing specialized knowledge across multiple areas of medicine and science as they relate to the work of dementia prevention. The philosophy and method that you will review in this work are the results of that organized effort. Successful dementia prevention requires a detailed understanding of concepts and principles in the specialties of cardiology, vascular medicine, rheumatology, hematology, oncology, sleep medicine, psychiatry, immunology, neuropathology, neuroradiology, pediatrics, internal medicine, infectious disease, genetics, electrophysiology, neuropsychiatry, and biochemistry. While physicians and providers of health care who dedicate their time to a single branch of medicine will have a much broader understanding of their specific field of study, the dementia prevention specialist coalesces all the facts that are important to how the brain is damaged and the effects of that damage to the brain and mind.

Using common sense and understanding of the concepts that I describe—rather than relying upon guidelines presented by others—will lead to successful results in the prevention of Alzheimer's disease and dementia. Guidelines are not always completed with accurate thought. Guidelines may be used where one cannot provide accurate thought to the current situation. Facts can change rapidly, yet principles will always hold true. A principle based upon experience and knowledge will reflect wisdom into decisions. Those working to the best of their ability may not have resources or knowledge of a specific subject, and falling back upon a guideline may be better than other options. Following a guideline requires no accurate thought—it allows individuals to know very little about the concepts and the principles behind what they are basing their decisions on. I do not allow others to do my thinking for me—it is better for one to review all of the facts and come to one's own conclusions.

As an individual seeking prevention of dementia, you must consider and be familiar with each individual aspect of dementia prevention to obtain your goal. You will be in a much better position to make decisions based on your unique needs once you understand the causes of dementia. Once you understand specific and detailed aspects of anatomy and physiology, you will be the best advocate for the prevention of your dementia. You will be your own individual expert, and as this expert, you will seek opinions from well-known institutions. You will then know if the advice you are receiving is based upon accurate thinking and common sense or based upon other factors. If you are a family member reading this work as part of the search to help a loved one, you are now one step closer to success.

Alzheimer's disease and dementia occur in a damaged brain. As there has never been a case of dementia that did not result from brain damage, one needs to understand all of the factors that can cause brain damage. The following will explore many reasons for damage to the brain. You or your loved one may have a single cause or a compounded case caused by multiple factors during the same time. Considering a unique individual, one factor could weigh more heavily than any other. Some cases can also be a compounded effect of different factors during different times of life, coming together in a perfect storm of mind damage.

CHAPTER 1

Causes of Brain Damage That Lead to Alzheimer's

Many current authors and scientists will rely upon field assumptions—areas of interest that may not have been proven or worked out yet—to try to move forward assumptions made by a group. "Widely assumed in the field" are not words that are based upon accurate thought; they simply describe concepts that have not been proven. One needs to proceed carefully as at times one's assumption may be based upon a prior assumption, and before you know it, almost everyone believes that the world is flat or the earth is the center of the universe. Understanding and challenging these assumptions can often result in direct conflict with what you already know, what you have read, or what others have told you. Some of what I will review here will work hand in hand with what others have told you and what you have read. Some aspects of this information have been well-proven and established in the medical literature.

I am a doctor; however, I am not *your* doctor. You need to get your health-care advice from your health-care team. I am here to provide you with medical information. This medical information will stimulate your conversations with your health-care team. In general, once a question is asked, it results in better care of the patient. Being a well-informed individual will help with your prevention of dementia. Current health care often bases guidelines on lack of evidence, rather than evidence against. Population patterns may be used, rather than scientific information and common sense. Guidelines designed to cover the masses may not apply to your needs. Evaluation of the individual's unique medical conditions allows for a halt in the further advances of memory and mind problems. This is also expanded into the reversal of dementia in some individuals. The reversal of dementia is clinically difficult to define. A growing number of anecdotal patients had professional neuropsychiatric scores that were completed, and then years later, when tested again, improved on their scores. Prospective clinical studies are under way to measure some exact details and publish the data.

The consequences of some medical conditions are so extreme that they need to be taken very seriously—even if there is only a small chance that they could result. Doing nothing at all to prevent dementia—or simply treating the symptoms—is going to end with dementia. The moment one is able to identify the cause(s) of brain damage, one is able to put the brakes on degradation and let the body heal. There is a general healing process in the brain; if you give it the opportunity to heal, you may discover that your memory and mind problems will improve.

We will briefly review a number of new concepts, such as cognitive conscious function (CCF), the micron stroke, and the idea that the brain does not age but is damaged over time. We will also describe in a more accurate way some existing issues, such as "senior moments," memory loss, and ministrokes or transient ischemic attacks (TIAs). These concepts were initially developed in the peer-reviewed journal article "The Micron Stroke Hypothesis of Alzheimer's Disease and Dementia" by A. J. Orehek, published in the May 2012 edition (volume 78, issue 5) of *Medical Hypotheses* (pp. 562–70). In the book *Prevention Is Difficult—But Possible* by Allen J. Orehek, MD, self-published in 2012 with CreateSpace

(ISBN 978-1475017526), I expanded on the method. These concepts have been formally presented internationally at various conferences, including the 2014 International Neuroscience Conference in Tokyo, Japan; Euroscicon's Alzheimer's Disease Congress in London in 2014; and the conference of the Spanish Neurology Society (Sociedad Espanola de Neurologia) Crystalline Tissular Network as part of the Morphofunctional Unit of the Central Nervous System in Valencia, Spain, in 2014. There is also a complete six-part video series on youtube.com/user/dementia-prevention entitled "Prevent Alzheimer's Disease" that provides information on this topic.

Micron stroke is a hypothesis used to describe damage to the brain so small that a single event is not noticed by the individual nor will it show up on any type of available scans (magnetic resonance imaging [MRI] or computerized tomography [CT]). This new scientific concept is different from silent cerebral ischemia and stroke, currently two ways to describe damage to the brain. It can take hundreds or thousands of micron-stroke events over time to damage a brain such that brain atrophy or brain age can be detected. The micron-stroke hypothesis indicates that very small damage can occur without one noticing it and without it being detected on an MRI. However, over time, the effects of micron strokes are devastating. Along with larger strokes, these are the reason for much brain atrophy, brain age, white matter changes, and the term *small vessel ischemic disease* that you will find filling radiology reports. This concept is also represented by the mathematical equation integrated into CCF.

Cognitive Conscious Function

There is much function of the brain that is beyond the medical field's current ability to comprehend, detect, study, grade, classify, evaluate, or score. One must appreciate that brain functionality is not just related to things that you can measure, judge, or understand. As a brain is damaged over time, one may experience a change in self-confidence or a difference in curiosity. These changes are very challenging to observe/measure even over decades. We do not have the technology, tools, or insight to understand even a fraction of what is the most complex structure in the known .. universe.

Most medical textbooks typically divide the brain into two general abilities: motor and sensory, sort of a general in and out of the brain function. CCF is a term to describe this powerhouse that is your brain. This term is used in the scientific equation that explains the prevention of dementia as published in "The Micron Stroke Hypothesis of Alzheimer's Disease and Dementia," *Medical Hypotheses* 78, no. 5 (2012): 562–70 (doi: 10.1016/j.mehy.2012.01.020) by A. J. Orehek. Higher functions are pooled into executive functions or higher-level reasoning, and yet even with detailed neuropsychiatric testing, only the surface of "you" is scratched. Stated in a slightly different way, one can observe unique individuals' interaction with the world through their senses, view how they move their body in response to intentional movements, and determine their ability to complete tests of memory and other functions, and yet we have no way to measure, judge, grade, or score their creativity. Here's another example: as a brain is damaged over time, one may experience a change in self-confidence or a difference in curiosity; as I noted above, these changes will be very challenging to observe or measure, even over decades. A final way to describe CCF is to consider the difference between behavior (measured, judged, graded, and scored) and thought (consciousness).

Sensory skills are the brain's ability to perceive and process stimuli. Consider that the same stimuli that your brain receives also allow the hands of the blind to read braille and provide the keen sense of vision to the sniper, the range of flavors to a wine taster, the expert nose to a perfumer, and the detailed hearing of a submarine sonar operator. Motor skills is the other general ability of the brain; this is what moves all your muscles. Consider that the same function as in your brain also moved the hand of da Vinci as he painted the *Mona Lisa*, gives dexterity to a neurosurgeon, allows flesh to be sculpted out of stone, controls the endurance of a marathon runner or mountain climber, and moves the muscles of the fastest sprinter. Your brain is made up of a hundred billion neurons—the same as the number of stars, one hundred billion, in our galaxy, the Milky Way. These hundred billion neurons are supported by a greater number of support cells, such as astrocytes, oligodendrocytes, microglia, vascular network, and glyphatic system. The number of potential connections in your brain is so tremendous that even astronomical numbers that deal with hundreds of millions or hundreds of billions still pale in comparison to the number of connections that you have in your own brain.

A BRIEF EXERCISE

Sensory and Motor

SENSORY

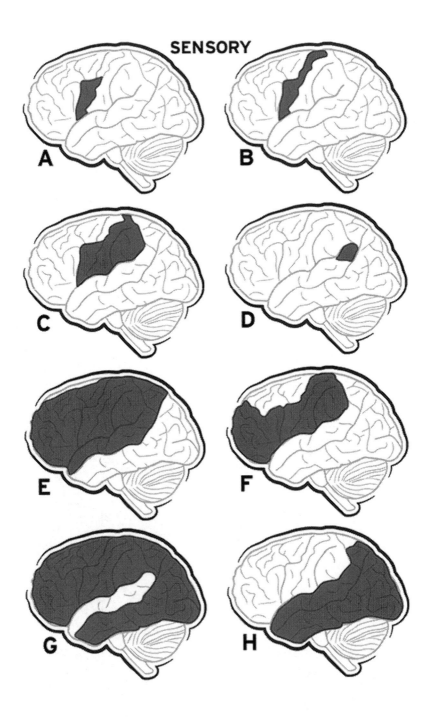

Sensory Question

Look at the two-dimensional images on the left. Decide for yourself how much of your brain is dedicated to the sensory system. How much of your brain is responsible for all of your ability to taste, touch, smell, hear, and see? The specific locations are not important, as some are not that well understood anyway; simply consider the area as related to the images. In this example each brain represents one hundred billion neurons. The shaded areas would be what you are trying to determine are used by your brain for your senses.

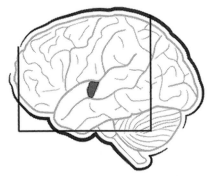

Few million neurons

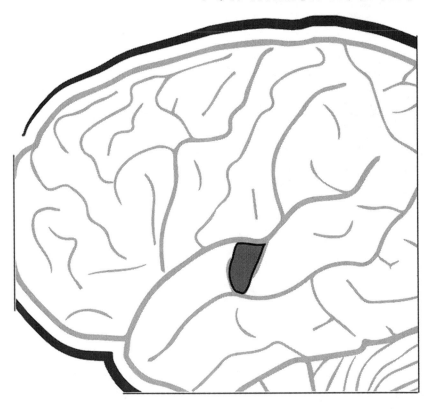

Sensory Answer

Answer: All of your senses are controlled by about one to two million cells. Consider that an adult butterfly also has five senses.

MOTOR

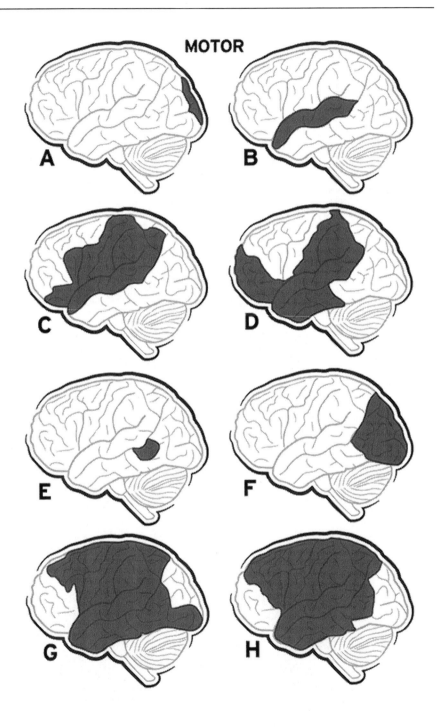

Motor Question

Look at the images on the left. Now, after knowing how much of your brain is committed to the sensory system, decide for yourself how much of your brain is dedicated to the motor system. How much of your brain is responsible for all of your ability to control all your movements and muscle actions?

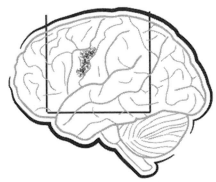

a few hundred thousand neurons

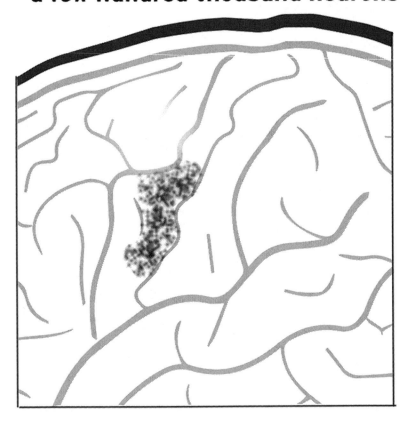

Motor Answer

Answer: Simply a few hundred thousand cells control all of your motor functions.

The important point here is that you visualize how much of your brain could be potentially damaged and you would never even know about it. Look at the known global functions of the brain and the aspects of the brain that are yet to be discovered. Take a brief look into the subconscious, and you will agree that much of the brain is yet to be discovered. Consider the brain to be likened to the ocean; we have only unlocked a swimming pool. We have a very long way to go in solving even the most basic mysteries of the brain. We spoke briefly of the two general abilities of the brain that most health-care teams attempt to judge, grade, score, or test. CCF is responsible for all of the functions of the brain that we discussed, plus your compassion, empathy, spirituality, insight, curiosity, and so on.

Micron Stroke

Micron stroke is a new scientific term defined in my paper "The Micron Stroke Hypothesis of Alzheimer's Disease and Dementia," mentioned above. When damage comes to the brain in general, your health-care team and medical textbooks currently will refer to this damage in three different ways. They will talk about a massive cerebral vascular accident (CVA), which is a big stroke; a TIA, which is considered a ministroke; and the silent cerebral ischemia. A fourth way that the brain can be damaged is from micron strokes.

Medical Hypotheses 78 (2012) 562–570

Contents lists available at SciVerse ScienceDirect

Medical Hypotheses

journal homepage: www.elsevier.com/locate/mehy

The Micron Stroke Hypothesis of Alzheimer's Disease and Dementia

Allen J. Orehek *

Dementia Prevention Centre™, 2637 E Atlantic Blvd #19129, Pompano Beach, FL 33062, United States

ARTICLE INFO

Article history:
Received 9 November 2011
Accepted 9 January 2012

ABSTRACT

Alzheimer's disease as currently described in the medical literature is often more a description of dementia rather than a specific disease. In over a century of scientific work there has been no proven theory as to the precise pathogenesis of Alzheimer's disease and dementia. As there is no efficient treatment for patients with Alzheimer's disease, prevention or attenuation of the disease is of substantial value.

An intricate collection of hypotheses, studies, research, and experience has made it complicated for one to completely understand this disease. The purpose of this hypothesis is to illustrate new concepts and work to link those concepts to the present understanding of an obscure disease. The search for a single unifying hypothesis on the etiology of Alzheimer's disease has been elusive. Many hypotheses associated to Alzheimer's disease have not survived the testing to become theory. Suggested here is that the elusive nature of etiology of dementia is not from one cause, but rather the causes are numerous.

Medical terminology used freely for decades is rarely evaluated in the light of a new hypothesis. At the foundation of this work is the suggestion of a new medical term: Micron Strokes.

The Micron Stroke Hypothesis of Alzheimer's Disease and Dementia include primary and secondary factors. The primary factors can be briefly described as baseline brain tissue, atrial fibrillation, hypercoagulable state, LDL, carotid artery stenosis, tobacco exposure, hypertension diabetes mellitus, and the presence of systemic inflammation. Dozens of secondary factors contribute to the development of dementia. Most dementia is caused by nine primary categories of factors as they interact to cause micron strokes to the brain.

© 2012 Elsevier Ltd. All rights reserved.

Introduction

Described by Alois Alzheimer in 1906 and named by Emil Kraepelin in 1910, Alzheimer's disease lacks a universally accepted definition. The Consortium to Establish a Registry for Alzheimer's Disease (CERAD) in a series of papers attempted to describe different criteria that could assist in assigning a diagnosis [1,2]. In the United States it is calculated that Medicare will spend 11.4 trillion on the disease over the next few decades [3]. By the year 2050 the annual cost of a disease is estimated to be 1.08 trillion [4]. The disease process is not only expensive, but also associated with high mortality. The number of deaths due to Alzheimer's disease increased by 66 percent between 2000 and 2008. The baby boom population, as it ages, will add a significant number of demented if no changes are made to the rate of occurrence. In 2010 the hours of care by millions of unpaid caregivers and family members contributed a value of $202 billion [5]. Medicare payments for services to beneficiary with Alzheimer's disease and other dementias are almost three times higher than the non affected beneficiaries [6].

In the 1990s the original histological slides from the early work of Alois Alzheimer were evaluated. Alzheimer's first described case (Auguste D.) had atherosclerosis [7]. The second published case (Johann F.) from Alois Alzheimer was found to have numerous plaques but no neurofibrillary tangles [8]. Not identifying neurofibrillary tangles in the second published case of Alzheimer's own work confounds the situation. Currently there is no clear understanding of the pathogenesis of Alzheimer's disease [9]. In reality the findings of neurofibrillary tangles and amyloid plaques in Alzheimer's disease might be independent of each other [10]. Other works have described details of the confusing history of dementia, including Alzheimer's Dementia. Some literature has developed sub-classes of Alzheimer's disease to assist in trying to describe their findings (e.g. sporadic, early onset, mixed). Often wherever one reads, they will discover vague and contradicting explanations of such a significant disease.

As related to this work the concept that micron strokes over time result in what is more generally referred to as "the normal ageing process of the brain." Micron strokes result in white matter changes. The majority of brain age process is due to recurrent insults by micron strokes over time. A flaw of CERAD is that they make the assumption that the brain has an ageing process. This work will challenge the 'normal ageing' of the brain by suggestion of an equation that describes the changes that occur in the brain over time (see "Concepts" section). This equation will also describe why so many studies find changes that occur over time, and end up considering these important findings to be part of a natural process. No doubt the final determination of all factors that cause

* Tel.: +1 516 986 7533.
E-mail address: reprint@micronstroke.com

0306-9877/$ - see front matter © 2012 Elsevier Ltd. All rights reserved.
doi:10.1016/j.mehy.2012.01.020

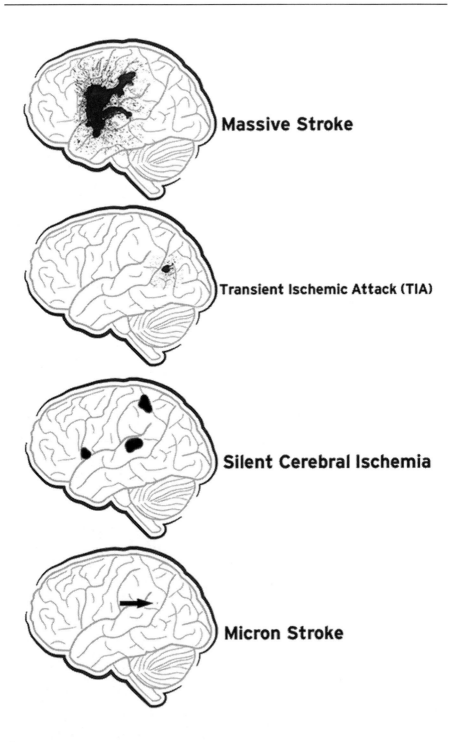

Massive Stroke

Transient Ischemic Attack (TIA)

Silent Cerebral Ischemia

Micron Stroke

A massive stroke is when there is sudden damage to the brain so extreme that you lose function of your body or abilities. CVA is damage to a large part of the brain, with the loss of many neurons. CVAs occur in many ways. Sometimes there is recovery as the brain works around the damaged areas; however, the dead neurons and cells will not come back. The brain has other networks that will start to help "heal" in a limited way. Some functions may return and appear normal despite the death of millions or hundreds of millions of brain neurons. Considering CCF, one will recall that there were many other aspects of the unique individual lost forever.

Transient ischemic attack or ministroke has many different descriptions. Committees sit down and try to come up with a proper way to describe this concept. In general, most medical textbooks and your current health-care team will refer to a ministroke or TIA as an occluded blood vessel (event) that then reopens and neurological function is restored. Sometimes the neurological deficits of a ministroke can last for minutes or an hour, but in general will last less than twenty-four hours. Imaging studies that are completed will be summarized by the radiology team as a "negative study," meaning they did not see massive damage. Later reviewers of the MRIs may note that there was brain damage, but the challenge to the current definitions of TIA is that the accurate facts do not add up. One cannot determine what was permanent damage that the brain was able to work around versus what was an occluded blood vessel that reopened, restoring neurological function. We will come back to this later.

Silent cerebral ischemia is where there is damage to the brain that is found on a scan. Some people may have been injured for a different reason—maybe they got in a car accident—and a scan of the brain was done, and the damage was noted unrelated to the reason for the scan. These people had no idea that they had any damage to their brains; they never knew that they had a stroke. When this scenario was studied in the scientific literature, they were able to find strokes as large as three centimeters—thirty thousand microns, the size of an egg yolk. These are brains that have had a significant amount of damage and the individual had no idea of the event.

A micron stroke provides damage to the brain so small that you never knew it happened and an imaging study of the brain will not show it. It will not be picked up in the singles or in the tens or even in the hundreds, but only as you start to approach thousands or many thousands of micron strokes. The damage to the brain is going to be very easy to pick up. Visit www.youtube.com/user/dementiaprevention for an animation of a micron stroke causing damage to neurons.

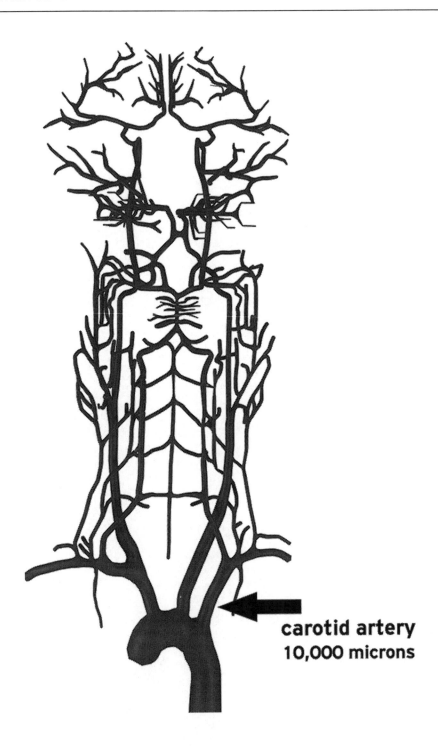

carotid artery
10,000 microns

This illustration represents the arteries that deliver blood from the heart to the brain. Some individuals will have an operation on the carotid artery due to cholesterol blockages. The largest arteries are your carotids, so large you can feel your pulse in your neck when blood is pumping through them.

To put a micron stroke into perspective, each carotid artery can have a diameter up to about ten thousand microns. These are the largest arteries, which go up through your neck into the brain.

The facing illustration takes us one step closer to understanding the size of a micron stroke. Many major named arteries are two thousand to five thousand microns in size. Often these arteries will be involved in a classic presentation of a major stroke due to the area of the brain that they deliver blood to. At times these arteries will also be used by interventional radiology teams to fix aneurysms.

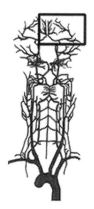

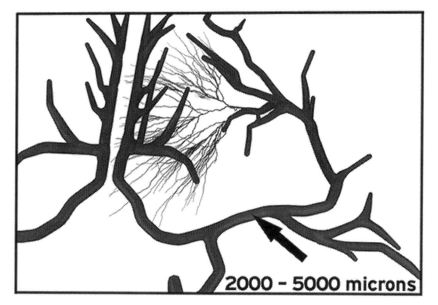

2000 - 5000 microns

Medium size arteries range from three hundred microns, while small arteries in the brain are one hundred microns or less. While not commonly named, some medium arteries may have names. Arteries of medium and small size vary greatly in location from individual to individual. Small arteries as shown here will not generally be named.

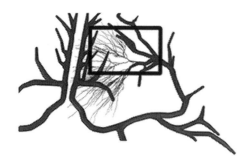

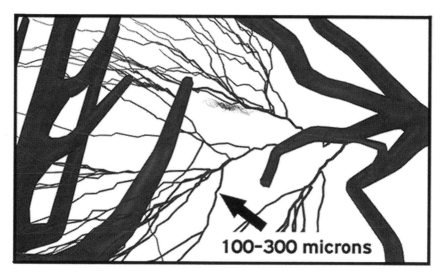

100-300 microns

Arteries smaller than one hundred microns branch out into even smaller thirty- to fifty-micron-size vessels.

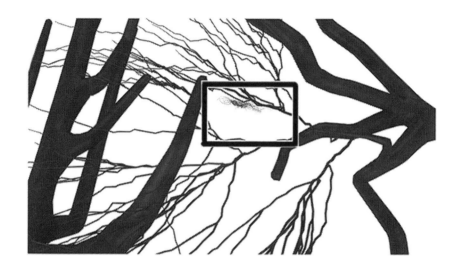

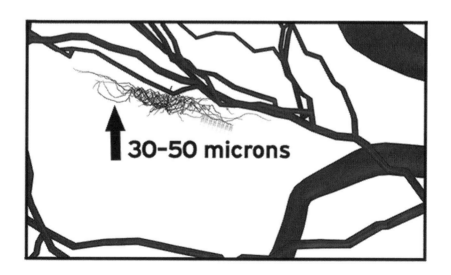

30-50 microns

The smallest arteries become what are known as arterioles, and their diameter is twenty to thirty microns. The walls of arterioles are thinner than those of arteries.

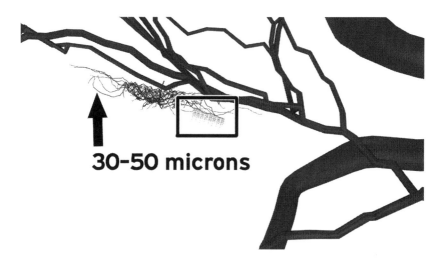

30-50 microns

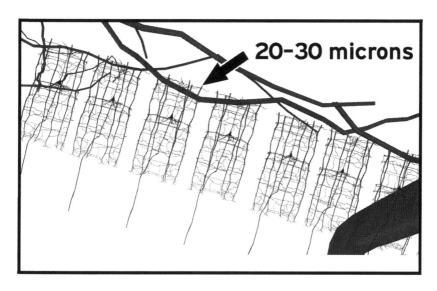

20-30 microns

This illustration shows the capillaries as part of the functional unit of the central nervous system. Capillaries are the smallest blood vessels. To the center of this "cage" of arterioles and capillaries, you will find the neuron. Recall that you have one hundred billion neurons. Now you can get an idea of where they are located. Each functional unit is estimated to contain fifty to one hundred neurons. This functional unit created of capillaries and arterioles is where your red blood cells and blood plasma provide oxygen and nutrients to your brain tissue. The width of a single red blood cell is about eight microns, and red blood cells pass through capillaries not much larger. The estimated length of just the capillaries is about four hundred miles—the distance from Washington, DC, to Boston. This capillary network provides one hundred square feet of surface area for interactions that supply nutrients. Each functional unit is located in a specific area of your brain; disruption of the blood supply to that unit damages it.

You can find an animated three-dimensional model of the functional unit at youtube.com/user/dementiaprevention.

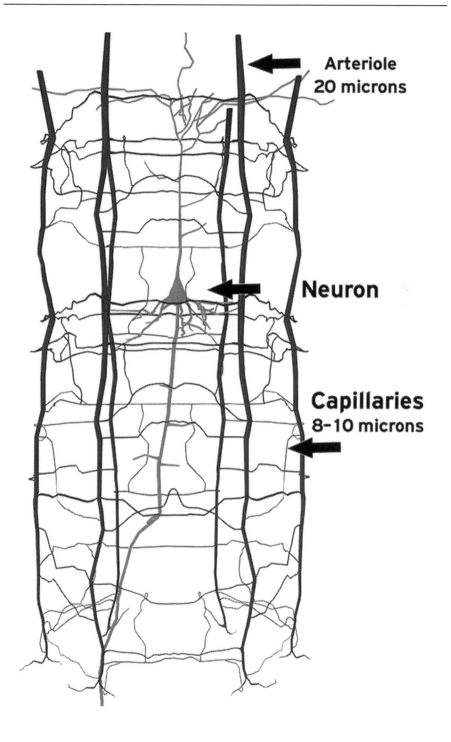

Arteriole
20 microns

Neuron

Capillaries
8-10 microns

An MRI of the Brain

The MRI is a loud banging machine that uses magnetic forces to detect differences in tissue properties without exposing you to radiation. Currently a 3-Tesla MRI will give you "slices" of the brain one thousand microns thick and space them about four thousand to ten thousand microns apart.

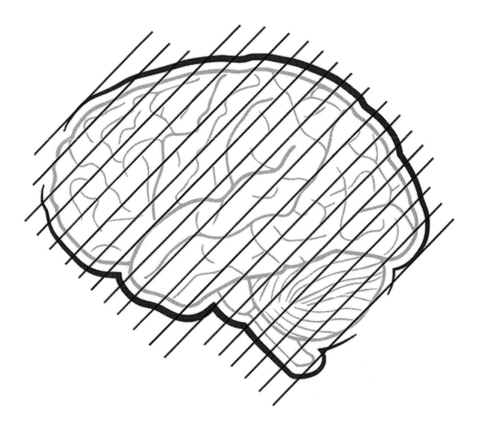

Once the images are computerized, they appear on a video monitor. The slices are an average of the tissue that was imaged. Current 3-Tesla MRIs can see damage in an area down to about one thousand microns. The MRI will not detect a static change at less than one thousand microns.

As the slices are usually obtained from five thousand to ten thousand microns apart, the brain tissue and neurons in the spaces between slices will go unevaluated. As a tool, the MRI will evaluate a volume of tissue, but not all of it. Computers are used to arrange texture and images from the MRI information, providing rather excellent landscape and general patterns of what the condition of your brain is. Blocked and injured arteries of one hundred or three hundred microns in size are unlikely to be detected. When a brain has suffered damage of one thousand to two thousand microns, this will be detected on the MRI as a small spot. Many radiology teams will ignore something of this size. These are considered small and unknown. Small spots such as these from one thousand micron-size strokes have not been well studied, and radiology teams are unsure of what effects they may have on your mind. Damage five thousand microns and less may be excluded when a scientific study that is looking at the amount of damage to the brain is completed or they are looking at strokes. Damage to the brain five thousand microns and more will be noted, but what term it will be given will vary from team to team (e.g., small stroke, white matter changes, punctuate lesions, multiple sclerosis, nonspecific demyelination, age-related brain changes, chronic small vessel ischemic disease, diffuse changes, age-appropriate changes, etc.).

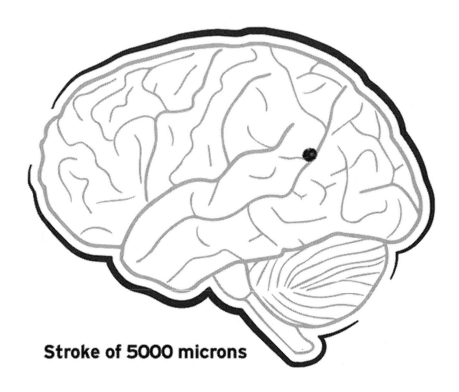

Stroke of 5000 microns

This illustration shows a five thousand micron-size area of damage to a brain. As you compare the size of the damaged area to the whole brain, you're able to see that even though this is a small stroke, a significant amount of damage to the brain could have occurred. (Millions of brain cells are dead.)

If one were to try to see a micron stroke by MRI, what would happen is that in making a comparison of an MRI before damage and an MRI after damage, the part of the brain will look the same because the micron stroke will be too small to be detected as a single event. For your consideration is the fact that micron strokes of ten to one hundred microns in size will be undetected; you may not know it happened, and your MRI team will not be able to identify the event. Damage has been done, cells have been killed, the cleanup process is under way, and the brain is rerouting living electric connections to provide you the best possible experience.

Reviewing this concept from a different perspective, the following illustrations describe the most important aspects of the morphofunctional unit as part of your brain. A review of this is important in understanding how a micron stroke can damage a small part of the brain and yet go unnoticed.

The illustration on the cover is an example of normal functional unit. This is a functional unit of the central nervous system as presented in the abstract of "The Crystalline Tissular Network of the Cerebral Cortex as the Functional Unit of the Nervous System" by Allen Orehek, José Rafael Iglesias-Rozas, Manuel Garrosa, and Carlos Esparza Sánchez.

The following pages illustrate how the many individual structures (cell types) come together to form the important functional unit. The functional units join together to create the crystalline network of the central nervous system. You will find that the final unit is made up of neuron, oligodendrocyte, capillary network, astrocyte, microglia, and interstitial fluid.

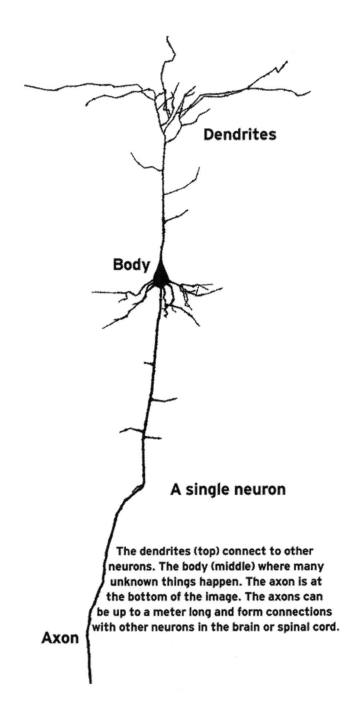

Dendrites

Body

A single neuron

The dendrites (top) connect to other
neurons. The body (middle) where many
unknown things happen. The axon is at
the bottom of the image. The axons can
be up to a meter long and form connections
with other neurons in the brain or spinal cord.

Axon

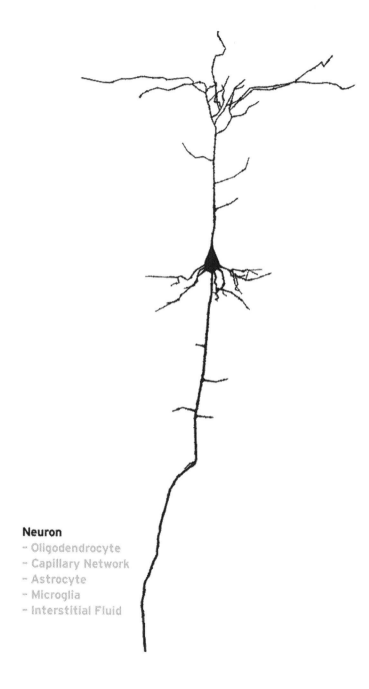

Neuron
- Oligodendrocyte
- Capillary Network
- Astrocyte
- Microglia
- Interstitial Fluid

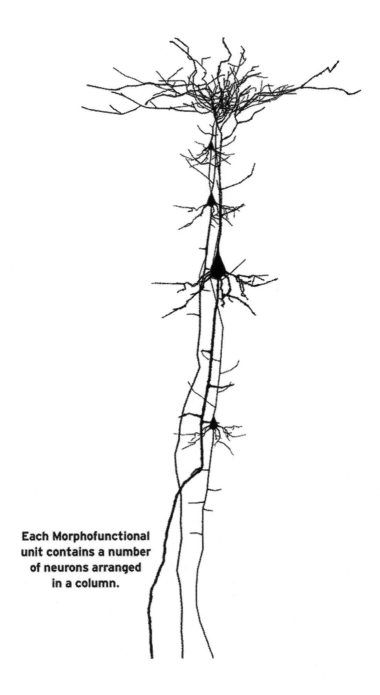

Each Morphofunctional
unit contains a number
of neurons arranged
in a column.

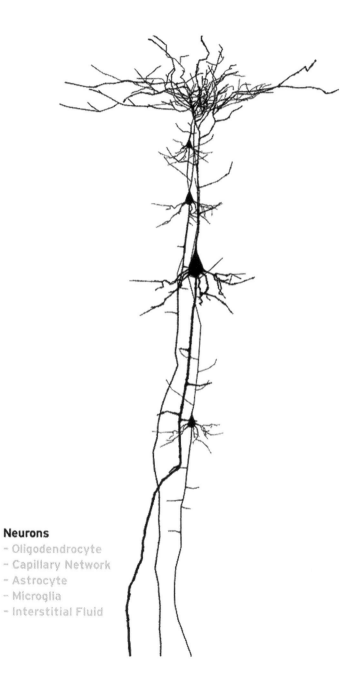

Neurons
- Oligodendrocyte
- Capillary Network
- Astrocyte
- Microglia
- Interstitial Fluid

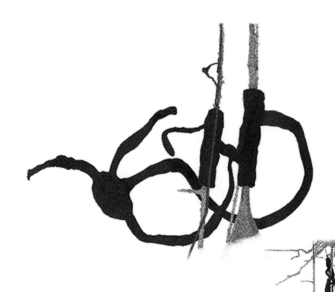

Oligodendrocytes

These brain cells have a special ability
to form insulating wraps around the neurons.
The oligodendorcytes come in many shapes
and sizes. By wrapping projections around
the neuron - the oligodendrocyte supports and
protects. Loaded with microtubules and
Tau proteins - when damaged they add to a
scar - (neurofibrillary tangle)

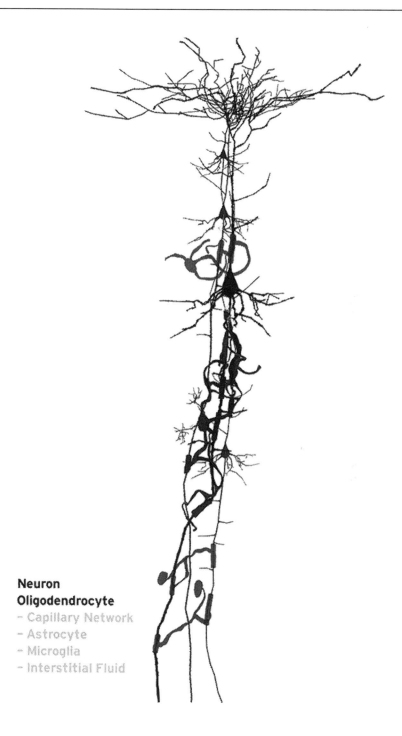

Neuron
Oligodendrocyte
- Capillary Network
- Astrocyte
- Microglia
- Interstitial Fluid

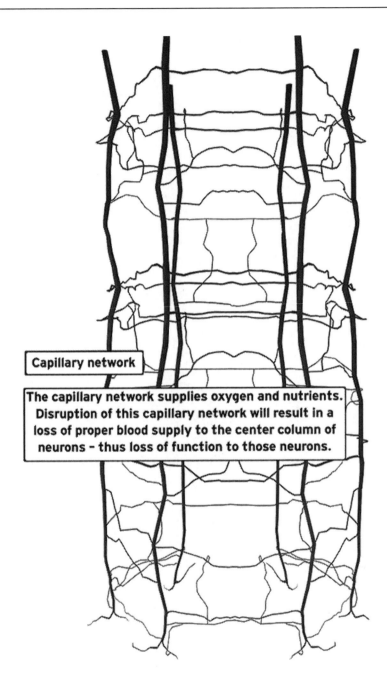

Capillary network

The capillary network supplies oxygen and nutrients. Disruption of this capillary network will result in a loss of proper blood supply to the center column of neurons - thus loss of function to those neurons.

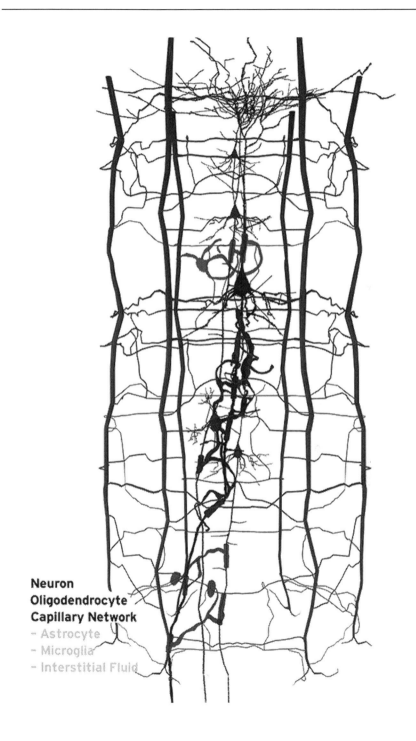

Neuron
Oligodendrocyte
Capillary Network
- Astrocyte
- Microglia
- Interstitial Fluid

Astrocytes

Astrocytes are specalized brain cells that connect
the capillaries with the neurons. They transport the
life giving nutrients - oxygen - proteins that help the
neuron function properly. Without the astrocytes the
neuron would die. The astrocytes form what is known
as the blood brain barrier. The astrocytes also regulate
the interstitial fluid, part of the glypahtic system.

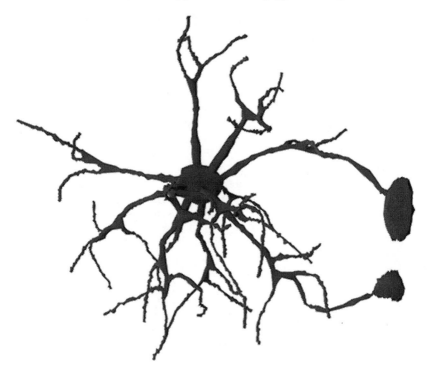

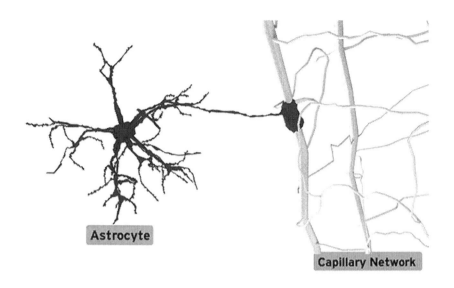

Astrocyte

Capillary Network

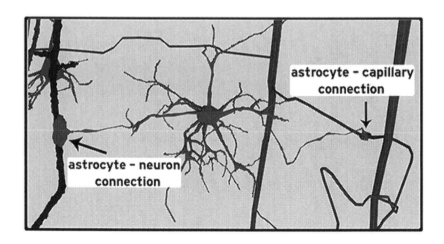

astrocyte – capillary connection

astrocyte – neuron connection

Astrocytes

Astrocytes are arranged in a specific geometric way. They are located in a pattern similar to the corners of a soccer ball. (icosahedron)

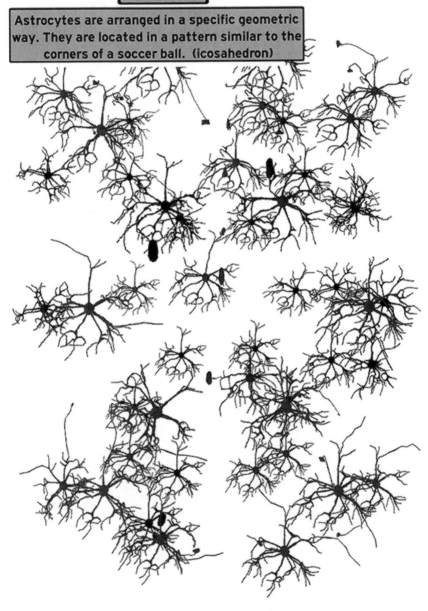

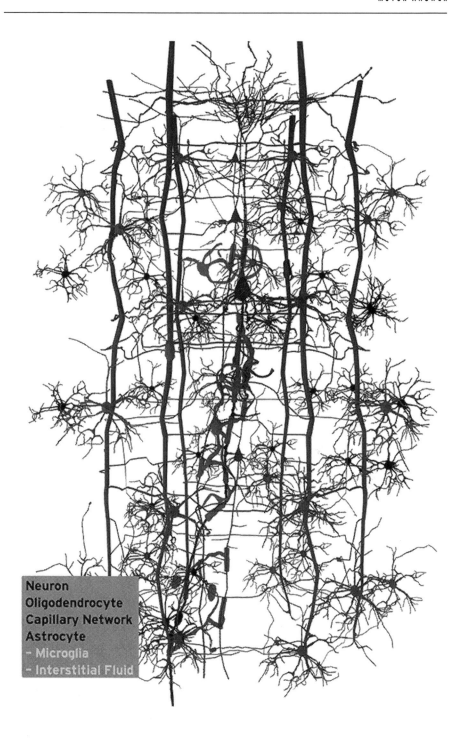

Neuron
Oligodendrocyte
Capillary Network
Astrocyte
- Microglia
- Interstitial Fluid

Microglia

Microglia are the scavengers in the brain tissue. These cells are spread throughout the nervous system and act to target infections and foreign material. Microglia can change their role and function as needed. They are able to respond to any need to fight inflammation or infection rapidly. They are able to produce many chemicals that assist in brain health, including production of amyloid precursor protein.

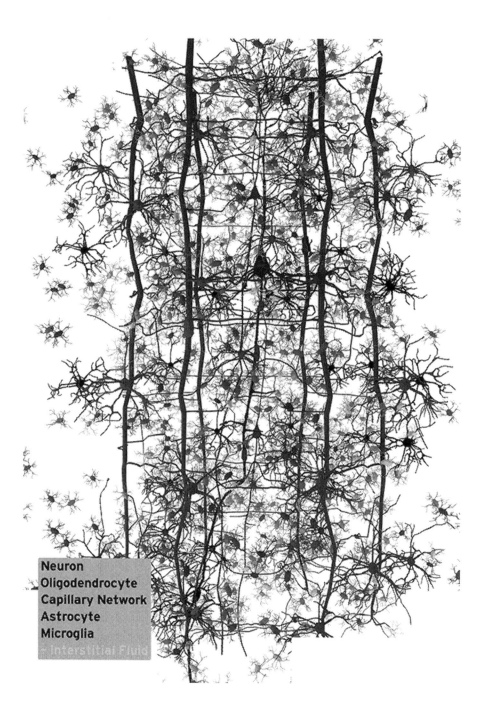

Neuron
Oligodendrocyte
Capillary Network
Astrocyte
Microglia
Interstitial Fluid

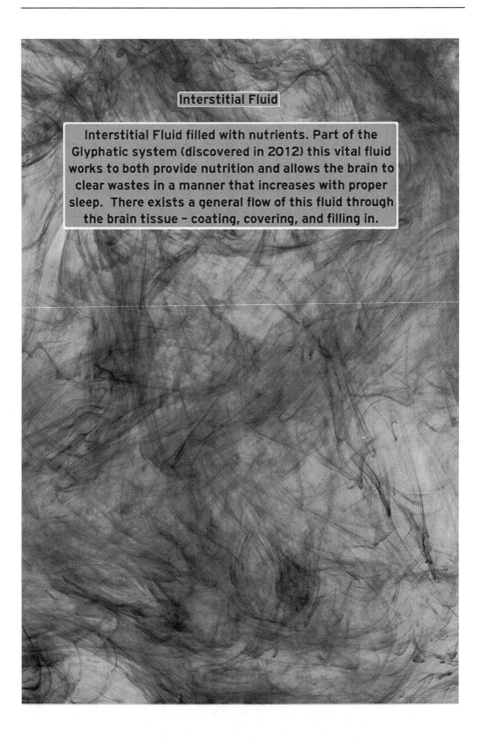

Interstitial Fluid

Interstitial Fluid filled with nutrients. Part of the
Glyphatic system (discovered in 2012) this vital fluid
works to both provide nutrition and allows the brain to
clear wastes in a manner that increases with proper
sleep. There exists a general flow of this fluid through
the brain tissue - coating, covering, and filling in.

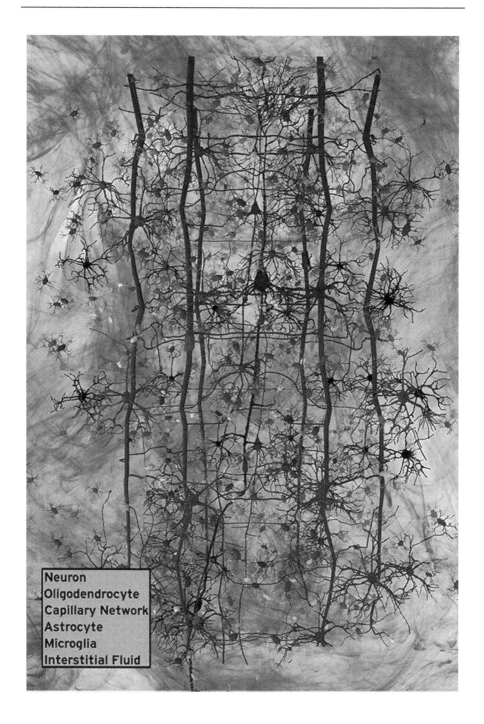

Neuron
Oligodendrocyte
Capillary Network
Astrocyte
Microglia
Interstitial Fluid

Each morphofunctional unit is organized into a geometric shape. Using the illustration of this shape one can visualize how the structure of the brain can reveal many details of how problems with mind and memory can start. (Example: Micron Stroke can damage a single unit and you will be unaware)

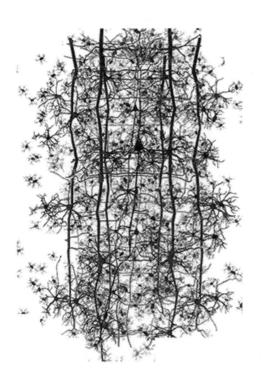
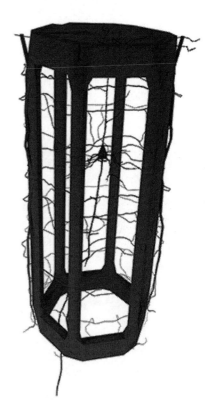

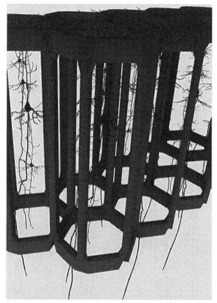

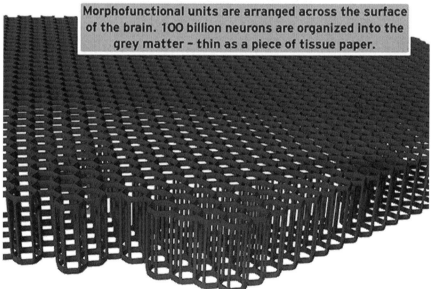

Morphofunctional units are arranged across the surface of the brain. 100 billion neurons are organized into the grey matter – thin as a piece of tissue paper.

You were just shown how one of the most important structures inside your brain is set up. This is where a number of specific cell types are doing very specific biological duties in support of the most important neuron. (In a car, it is the engine; in the kitchen, it is the stove; for your computer, it is the keyboard; and for a city, it is the power grid.) Without the proper function of the neuron, your functional unit will not be performing as expected; and if dead, the neurofibrillary tangle will be a monument that represents an old battlefield. With normal blood flow into the arterioles and capillaries, the astrocytes are able to take up fresh nutrients and supply them to the neuron, providing for its every need. This is the normal function.

The illustration is an example that attempts to explain the "widely accepted in the field" concept of TIA (ministroke). TIA is often defined as, "an occluded blood vessel reopens, and neurologic function is restored."

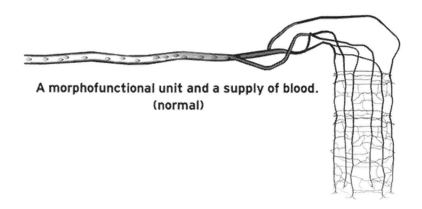

A morphofunctional unit and a supply of blood.
(normal)

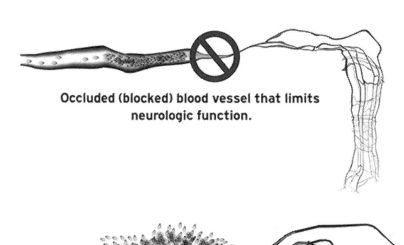

Occluded (blocked) blood vessel that limits
neurologic function.

"Accepted" concept of a Mini-Stroke (TIA). An
occluded blood vessel reopens restoring
neurologic funtion.

As mentioned before, I find it very unlikely that an artery or capillary in the brain can be occluded and then within a matter of minutes or an hour reopen. Arteries in the body don't work that way. Take, for example, blood clots. A partial evaluation of the known coagulation cascade, as illustrated below,

Coagulation Cascade

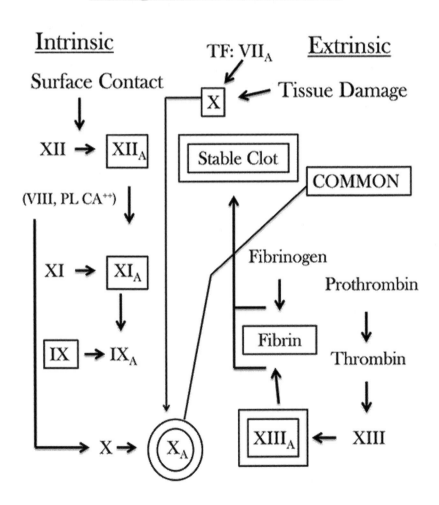

shows how your body forms clots or has the ability to block off a blood vessel; this clearly shows you that it is very difficult for a stable clot to do anything other than be a stable clot. Without clots you could bleed endlessly from a minor cut, so the clotting system is very useful and vital. At times clots form where we do not want them. When people have a clot that goes to the heart (specifically an artery that feeds the heart), it's considered a heart attack. People who have a heart attack go to a heart cauterization lab or someone who uses a clot-buster medication to open that artery. If the artery is not opened, then part of the heart dies; this is a heart attack or myocardial infarction (MI). These arteries don't spontaneously reopen.

Thinking of the "widely accepted" concept of TIA in the same light, it would almost seem strange that an occluded blood vessel in the brain would spontaneously reopen in a matter of minutes or less than an hour. The equivalent would be that you actually have to go to the cardiac catheterization lab and do some type of a balloon or intervention to get an artery to open up or be able to administer some type of a medication that would break the clot. One should consider that the brain might have a different, alternative way of restoring neurologic function after an artery is occluded.

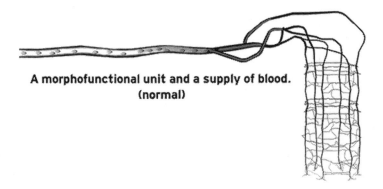

A morphofunctional unit and a supply of blood.
(normal)

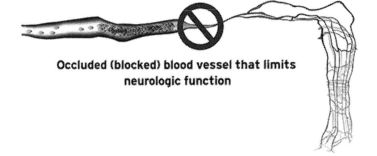

Occluded (blocked) blood vessel that limits
neurologic function

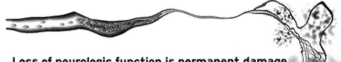

Loss of neurologic function is permanent damage
to morphofunctional units of the brain – with
function being restored after the
brain makes adjustments.

A reasonable explanation for the same events is that once the oc-cluded blood vessel occurs, the neurological function is disturbed for a period of time, whether it's minutes or an hour, but the dam-age is permanent to the affected functional units.

The brain is able to reroute, recalculate, and make adjustments. We can witness this type of brain rerouting after massive strokes as the neurons reconnect and attempt to restore function. The brain is a very tricky thing, and it wants to be able to restore that func-tion. So in the end, the neurological function is restored, but it is not because a blood vessel reopened. This is significantly different from the current scientific literature and the medical textbooks. This has not been studied. If your health-care team views TIA as a blood vessel that was blocked and then reopened and restored neurological function, then the information used to treat you by your health-care team is not accurate.

I totally disagree that you are back to everything being blissful. I believe the damage was permanent, and over time all of these small areas that you may or may not notice are going to add up and give you "brain aging," along with memory and mind issues. When you're dealing with a concept that is evaluating the damage that a ten-micron stroke would cause to the brain over time, you will find that a signifi-cant amount of scientific research needs to be completed. Injury to the morphofunctional units as part of the crystalline cerebral network over time will result in neuron death and loss and all of a vast variety of events, such as healing, amyloid, and scar, which will follow in the wake of this damage. Consider a stroke to be a winter snowstorm; a micron stroke would be a single snowflake.

> The brain does not age, but it does
> take damage over time.

The brain does not age. As you get older, you develop better language skills; you increase your vocabulary; you're able to improve social and complex reasoning skills; your inductive reasoning improves; you practice an enhanced application of your trust; you're able to enjoy incorporating decades of experience into new decisions; spatial reasoning improves; you become better with your ability to focus more on positive information and less on the negative; and you enjoy enhanced wisdom. These abilities are not compatible with the decay of an organ. Biopsies from the brain of the most aged will show perfectly normal brain tissue (neurons) next to brain tissue damaged from micron strokes (and larger strokes). The concept that the brain does not age is significantly different from what you have been taught. This may also actually directly conflict with what you have learned.

Let me share. I love satellite learning programs. My DVR is filled with almost every type of learning program. While I was working on the Micron Stroke Hypothesis article mentioned above,

I was watching one such program. A renowned physicist came on, and he started to describe how everything in the universe can be explained by mathematical equations. He started to draw out equations for matter, energy, time, and space. How a glass of milk is able to remain on the counter can be simply explained by a mathematical equation. That is when it hit me: if I could describe the prevention of dementia with a mathematically correct equation, then I would have something that would be able to be offered to the world that could be weighed, measured, researched, and judged. This is my mathematical representation of why the brain does not age and how the presumed "aging" is related to damage over time.

$$CCF = CCF_O - \sum_{n=1}^{N} W_n * f_n(t)$$

CCF_O = initial conditions of cognative conscious function

N = The total number of insults (Example: micron strokes) acting in one individual (Includes the Primary and secondary categories)

W_n = Weighting of each risk factor

$f_n(t)$ = The shape function that describes effect of micron stroke insult, potential recovery as a function of time.

The Dementia Prevention Center created a research project where MRI images were provided to radiology teams. They were not told the age of the brains. Without this information, they were unable to properly ascertain the age of an individual brain. A brain of a younger person that was damaged from micron strokes was viewed as that of a person decades older. The MRI of older individuals who protected their brains from the effects of micron strokes were viewed as those of individuals many decades younger. When the radiology teams did not know the age of a patient, they were unable to look at the MRI and say what was "age-appropriate" change to the brain. Reviewing MRI reports, if you see words such as *age-appropriate white matter changes*, the radiologist is making the assumption that the brain has a natural aging process. This is a general gestalt that has been handed down from older physicians as they train newer physicians. But an aging process inside the brain is not something that has ever been proven or established one way or the other.

An additional way to think of this is to consider the following: "If a sixty-five-year-old who protected his or her brain from the effects of micron strokes all those years had a normal brain, would this then actually be considered abnormal because there was no damage? Where there were no age-appropriate changes?" The radiology world simply cannot have it both ways. A normal brain that has been protected cannot all of a sudden be the abnormal brain. The abnormal brain that has suffered damage from decades of micron strokes cannot be considered normal. Simply because a problem is very common does not make it the normal state—and brain damage is very common.

One can consider that if there were a process of aging to the brain, then after some time, the MRI of the brain would be the same or similar in each person. Damage would be in a specific location and pattern due to "the way of things." If there was a process in the brain of ageing then when one looked at the MRI from ten individuals of the same age, you would see the same patterns. The configuration of damage and loss would be similar from individual to individual because of the process of aging. Consider as part of the Micron Stroke Hypothesis that there is no innate process; you see damage from different factors that should be evaluated in that individual. Damage occurring in different locations in different configurations in different individuals to different extents is compatible with the factors and etiology outlined in this work. The evaluation of a brain that has any degree of damage must be thorough and complete, as some causes may be rare.

CHAPTER 2

Steps to Accurate Alzheimer's Prevention

This chapter outlines a step-by-step program that may help you to prevent dementia. The full description of the method is a lengthy technical document, and that does not include an explanation of every medical term and every medical concept. The basis of what we will review is in Patent US 8708906 B1, "Method for the Prevention of Dementia and Alzheimer's Disease," filed on September 7, 2011, and published on April 29, 2014. Inventor: Allen J. Orehek.

I'm going to give you a direct shortcut to the prevention of dementia. You do not need to know exactly how your smartphone works in order to enjoy your piece of technology; you send an emoji or a text message to a friend, not understanding all of the computer codes, data transfers, cell towers, microwaves, and operating systems. These things are not important for you to be able to use and enjoy your technology. Consider that they are all facts, but not very important facts for you to know in the use of your technology. I'm going to be presenting to you the prevention of dementia in much the same way—without getting into all of the details.

Now, don't get me wrong. I'd love to sit and review all of the details with you; we could easily spend a couple hours. In fact, that's all that I do. People who know me know that this is my passion, my state of dharma. All I do is talk about this. So at some point in time, we can sit down, we can arrange research, we can talk about cases of success, and we can develop new concepts. That is not our goal for this chapter, though. Before we start, rather than continually explaining that accurate thought on a topic may differ significantly from the thought of your health-care team and academic guidelines, I will simply tell you to watch, understand, and choose what path works best for you. For some, following supplied guidelines from your health-care team works perfectly. It may be what you need. For others, who wish to prevent Alzheimer's disease and dementia, grab a pen and paper. Take notes. Leave comments.

Challenges:
For some who seek dementia prevention the initial challenges may be found in the current healthcare system. Those who have many complex medical problems, some of which have not been fully and accurately diagnosed, could struggle to get accurate information. Some providers of healthcare may not be able to adjust a fixed daily schedule to accommodate a patient with a significant amount of medical and technical data. You may need sixty five minutes of face to face discussion in a fifteen minute time slot. For this challenge you may need to become your own best expert, gathering your medical information and assisting in the integration. If your primary healthcare team is not able to manage the interactions of multiple medical conditions you may need to separate some conditions out into specialists.

Brain Images
First, you need to have a magnetic resonance imaging (MRI) of your brain (cash price circa 2016 is about $475), and it needs to be read properly. Remembering the part about the brain does not age, I explained what you will be looking for in a proper reading of your brain MRI. That may be a challenge. Here at the Dementia Prevention Center, we scrutinize the data that can be obtained from

an MRI, and the interpretation is made independent of the age of the client. An MRI tells how much damage your brain has suffered over time and serves as your baseline for future comparison.

Memory Testing

Second, you need to get neuropsychological testing completed the first year you have a senior moment. The test takes six hours; there are no shortcuts. For many this will serve as a baseline, but for a few it will also identify that there is already a problem with their cognitive conscience function (CCF). Recall my previous information on CCF and how it decreases over time based on the amount of damage the brain suffers. The priority in this step is for you to identify and understand your CCF independent of your health-care team, who may only pick its problems in the advanced stages. Many current health-care teams will use mini-mental state examination (MMSE)—a very quick test that will not accurately assist in determining your CCF. Your health-care team will use a less accurate tool in "nonobvious" cases because this tool is designed to be cost-effective and quick. Few things in dementia prevention will be quick, and yet all will be cost-effective if your goal is to continue to live at home and maintain your own mind.

Atrial Fibrillation

Third, as indicated here, the individual who is interested in dementia prevention will get an ultrasound of the heart (2-D echo circa 2016 is about $375). This study needs to next be read accurately for the details needed. Those details would contain the size of the left atrium and condition of all four valves. Following changes in size of the left atrium will allow an individual to be well prepared for any of the earliest days of atrial fibrillation (also called afib). Starting treatment at the first increase in size of the left atrium would also be a reasonable plan—and help you avoid the problem with atrial fibrillation altogether. Those who have atrial fibrillation and have not had it detected yet—or it has been detected and not mitigated—will have micron strokes every day. They will also have more massive strokes due to untreated/undertreated atrial fibrillation.

Atrial fibrillation is an abnormal quivering of a chamber of the heart. Many preventable factors can lead to atrial fibrillation. Once pressures in the heart change due to abnormal function of the heart valves, the sizes of the chambers start to change. Many stages of what becomes atrial fibrillation can be prevented or avoided if identified in advance. Very early stages (decades before) may present as some swelling in the legs. When patients present to a health-care team at a younger age with "just a bit" of swelling in the legs, they may be given a medication and no further evaluation, such as a complete cardiac and biochemical evaluation. One will find that contact with a physician of medicine who will look at the first identification of leg swelling as a sign indicating the start of a different problem is rare. There could be many causes of leg swelling, and at the top of the list is improper function of the heart or heart valves.

A short animation at www.youtube.com/users/dementiaprevent video afib will provide visual information to your understanding of atrial fibrillation.

Generally speaking, the function of the heart is to pump blood. This requires proper filling of the heart with blood and proper function of the valves. When valves are working properly, then blood is allowed to flow in the correct direction. Your heart has four valves. The right side of the heart has a pressure that is lower than the left side of the heart. With each heartbeat blood flows in, valves close, and then blood flows out in a direction different from where it came in. This pumping system works very well—as long as all of the structural components (valves and muscle) are working efficiently. At age eleven, each of the valves has opened and closed about five hundred million times.

> ## Five hundred million openings and closings by about eleven years of age

There is nothing subtle about how the valves are slammed together—this happens rapidly and with some force. Your creator did a wonderful job in the design of this part of your body. Nothing that is made by humans would ever be able to keep pace for such wear and tear over time. With your heart valves, it is simply a matter of time until wear and tear can be detected. In some individuals, significant problems may develop prior to age eleven—also known as an "innocent murmur." While some murmurs of the heart are, indeed, considered normal functions of that unique heart, without knowing the condition of the valves, the pressures, and the sizes of the chambers, one is taking a large risk with that quick visit to the health-care provider.

You need to know the size of the chambers of your heart. You need to know the detailed condition of the valves of your heart. Once your heart left atrium reaches forty millimeters, you are at risk for atrial fibrillation. At fifty millimeters, your risk of atrial fibrillation is extreme—or you have it already and are yet unaware. As valves may change over time due to wear and tear—affecting the pressure in each chamber—you may experience a change in the size of the chambers due to those changes.

Some atrial fibrillation will be detected when you have symptoms such as rapid heart rate, stroke, feeling unwell, feeling jittery, an internal quiver feeling, mild nausea, sick to the stomach, trouble breathing, some abdominal discomfort, or any of the other ways that atrial fibrillation can present once symptomatic. The trick here is detecting atrial fibrillation before you actually notice symptoms from it. This can be done with an electrocardiogram (EKG, an electrical tracing of the heart), an overnight monitor, an extended monitor, and loop recorders. If you're able to detect it and treat it before a stroke occurs, that is a big advantage to you. These are decisions you need to make. A clear understanding of the condition of the heart valves and the size of the chambers of the heart is mandatory to the prevention of Alzheimer's and to the prevention of dementia.

Should you be one who is dealing with atrial fibrillation, consider the use of testing to reduce or eliminate your chances of a bleeding complication. One who will have a properly performed colonoscopy (scope up the bottom) and esophogastroduodenoscopy (scope down the throat) will be able to eliminate or identify most medical conditions that would provide a proclivity to bleeding. If one needs a blood thinner, then it could be an advantage to know the condition of the stomach and lower gastrointestinal system as many future bleeding-type complications could be eliminated (e.g., Barrett's esophagitis, esophatitis, *Helocobacter*, gastritis, colon polyp, stomach ulcer, infection, arterial venous malformations, etc.).

Carotid Arteries

Fourth, you need to get an ultrasound of your carotid arteries. Carotid arteries provide most of the blood flow to your brain. They serve as a nidus (place of origination) for micron strokes and strokes. An ultrasound of these arteries (cash price circa 2016 is about $240) is relatively simple because the arteries are close to the surface. There is no radiation from this test, which is considered noninvasive. The ultrasound is the same technology that allows mothers to snap an image of their unborn child, using sound waves to look inside the body in real time. There are two very important trends in the reporting of the results of a carotid artery ultrasound—common and accurate. The common trend is not going to be very useful; you will be looking for a report with more accurate details. The vast majority of testing (common) will be interpreted and reported as a blockage in the neck that needs to go for surgery or not. With the common trend, the majority of ways this will be reported back to your health-care team is that the results will say you either need to have surgery on your neck or not, there is a big blockage or not. That is not good enough. A more accurate report will have the exact percentage of blockage in your neck, providing accurate information that you need. This is what the Dementia Prevention Center needs for the prevention of dementia: we need to know what percentage of blockage there is based on your age. If your report contains words such as *no significant carotid artery stenosis*, then you need to discard that report and try again. You may have to try a number of times until you can finally find a facility that will provide you a report of the exact percentage of blockage in your neck. It is either zero or a percentage. Animated versions of carotid artery disease can be found on our YouTube site: youtube.com/user/Dementiaprevention.

When you have your accurate report, you can make a comparison of your percentage of blockages to an animation at www.youtube.com/user/Dementiaprevention. You need to realize that any blockages you have are not simply located in the carotids, but rather, they are a reflection of the rest of the arteries in the brain. Take caution with the opinion of "not much to worry about" on your ultrasound report. The ultrasound is only able to see the very start of miles and miles of blood vessels going up into your brain supporting the mind.

As I said above, beware of the term *no significant carotid artery stenosis* that may appear in your report. Such a statement is not accurate; we are looking for an exact percentage of blockage. Realize that there are four arteries that supply blood flow to the brain. No one can determine when there has been a reduction in flow that is significant in any one single artery. You have three other arteries that are supplying blood flow at the same time. But to expand this point slightly, no one knows the difference between blockages of 50 percent that are on their way to 49 percent, compared to a blockage that is 50 percent on its way to 51 percent. The physiology of that localized area is totally different in the two situations.

If you do have blockages, do not lose hope. Here at the Dementia Prevention Center, we have successfully dissolved many blockages in the body with medical treatment (sometimes through medication even). All the attention is to the details, excruciating details. To our understanding, we are the only facility that has data on successfully dissolved blockages with medical treatment. We have studied this and plan to publish the data. The data will be considered observational, so it is very unlikely that it will ever reach any academic guidelines. Future funding will hopefully allow us to prepare accurate randomized controlled trials. Many of our success stories took more than five years.

Blood Pressure

Fifth, know your blood pressure. Simply put, keep your systolic blood pressure less than 119 throughout your life. Forget terms like *borderline, elevated, prehypertension, high-normal, hypertension stage 1, hypertension stage 2, severe high blood pressure,* and *hypertension stage 3.* Those are different codes and symbols that all represent the same problem—high blood pressure. If you have high blood pressure, get it treated. That may not be as simple as stated because when studied in the United States, most people with high blood pressure go untreated or undertreated.

When you start out on your quest for accurate treatment of blood pressure problems, be sure to request from the heath-care team the reason for the change in blood pressure. Examples are blocked arteries to the kidneys (renal artery), blocked artery to the heart muscle (coronary artery), blocked artery to the brain (carotid artery), sleep apnea, poor choice in some social habits, poor function of heart valves, moderate damage to organs that is yet unknown, tumors (benign and cancerous), or a wide variety of more rare metabolic or endocrine disorders. Be sure to evaluate and treat the underlying reason for the blood pressure elevation, and then look for your dementia prevention goals. Proceed carefully if you are simply given a medication and placed into a risk guideline without understanding why your pressure is elevated.

For further reading on blood pressure goals and the science behind them, consider the following articles:

Rapsomaniki, Eleni, Adam Timmis, Julie George, Mar Pujades-Rodriguez, Anoop D. Shah, Spiros Denaxas, Ian R. White, Mark J. Caulfield, John E. Deanfield, Liam Smeeth, Bryan Williams, Aroon Hingorani, and Harry Hemingway. "Blood Pressure and Incidence of Twelve Cardiovascular Diseases: Lifetime Risks, Healthy Life-Years Lost, and Age-Specific Associations in 1.25 Million People." *The Lancet* 383, no. 9932 (2014): 1899–1911.

Dawber, Thomas R., Gilcin F. Meadors, Felix E. Moore Jr., National Heart Institute, National Institutes of Health, Public Health Service, Federal Security Agency, Washington, DC. "Epidemiological Approaches to Heart Disease: The Framingham Study." Paper presented at a Joint Session of the Epidemiology, Health Officers, Medical Care, and Statistics Sections of the American Public Health Association, the Seventy-Eighth Annual Meeting, St. Louis, MO, November 3, 1950.

Wright, J. T., L. J. Fine, D. T. Lackland, G. Ogedegbe, and C. R. Dennison Himmelfarb. "Evidence Supporting a Systolic Blood Pressure Goal of Less than 150 mm Hg in Patients Aged 60 Years or Older: The Minority View." *Annals of Internal Medicine* 160 (2014): 499–503. doi:10.7326/M13–2981.

> Lack of evidence is not the same as evidence against...

Diabetic?

Sixth, know your average blood sugar level. If you have type 1 or type 2 diabetes, get your three-month average. Do your best to keep your glyclohemoglobin (HgA1c) under 6.5. The closer to 6.0, the better for you. Anything over 6.5 is allowing additional damage to be done to your brain (and other tissues). For those who are diabetic but unsure if they are a type 1 or a type 2, a blood test called the C-peptide will allow you to know the function of your pancreas. Should you have a pancreas that is still producing insulin naturally, then dietary changes, lifestyle changes, and medications may help you get to your goal without the need of insulin. Many people will find the loss of five or ten pounds of body weight to be the difference between being diabetic and not being diabetic.

LDL Cholesterol

Seventh, know your cholesterol levels. Be warned: what I describe here will directly conflict with some of the most recent published academic guidelines. The main difference is that the published academic guidelines never look at the carotid arteries. In fact, many academic institutions recommend against looking at the carotid arteries until there are symptoms. You understand that symptoms may not always come until the more advanced stages of a problem. If you had a properly performed carotid artery ultrasound, then you know the condition of your carotid arteries. If there is a blockage in your carotid arteries, get your LDL cholesterol between 50 and 70. If your carotid arteries are clear—there are zero blockages—then keep your LDL cholesterol less than 100 through your life. If at any point your LDL cholesterol is over 100, you are simply adding blockages to your body. Now, if your genetic code is bad or you are a person who has extremely high LDLs, then you may need lipophoresis. These are terms that you will not necessarily see presented to you with academic guidelines, but these are things that exist in medicine and science and they can be offered to you to help get your LDL cholesterol down to where it needs to be. Even if you decide not to avail yourself of lipophoresis, consider that you at least were afforded the choice and your decision was to allow the cholesterol to remain high; this is different from never being provided any options.

When your LDL is over 100, you will be developing blockages. The higher your number, the faster you will be developing these blockages. While this is a crossroads of academic opinions, many physicians of medicine and providers of medical care will agree.

Providers of health care may simply follow whatever guidelines are placed in front of them. This then becomes your dilemma. We at the Dementia Prevention Center have successfully dissolved blockages in the human body by adding this method to a wider method of care for a unique individual.

Guidelines will usually look at the carotid arteries once you have symptoms. This point always confuses me. Those who write academic guidelines about the condition of the carotid arteries would probably not sign their name to a similar guideline that said wait for high blood pressure to have symptoms before you identify or treat it, or wait for there to be symptoms in a diabetic before you would identify it or treat it. So common sense demands that when a stroke is something preventable, when dementia is something that is preventable, knowing the condition of your carotid arteries would be of big benefit.

Tobacco

Eighth, do not smoke. If you're using tobacco, you must stop. The chemicals in the tobacco will cause your platelets (blood cells) to stick together and form small clots. The tobacco will also cause physiologic problems to the lining of the blood vessels that injure them and cause locations for damage and buildups. Those who cannot quit or are exposed to second hand smoke will have micron strokes on a daily basis. For those who are unable to quit, then considering the per-puff effect on the body may help you to cut back on the number of puffs you take each day. Think of your tobacco use as a per-puff and attempt to take even fewer puffs per cigarette. Should this be a problem for you, then your attention across all other primary categories is even more critical.

Sleep Apnea or Poor Sleep

Ninth, get a good night's sleep. Often people will simply say that they can fall asleep at any time during the day—or have fatigue that will not go away. Often people who have such issues will present to their health-care team with such a complaint, perhaps some labs will be drawn, they'll be given some reassurance and advice on proper exercise, and yet the important test of the polysmography will not be ordered.

The polysmography is a simple test (circa 2016 the cost is about $375). For this test, you will go and sleep in a sleep lab for a night. You will be hooked up to a number of monitoring devices that will evaluate your sleep. The evaluation generally includes stages of sleep, rapid eye movement (REM) sleep, heart rate, respiration rate, and oxygen levels. All of the details from a properly completed sleep study will be used to be sure you are getting proper sleep. The discovery of the brain's glyphatic system in 2012 has increasingly made the use of daily proper sleep very important. Early understanding of the brain's glyphatic system is that a significant increase in efficiency occurs when you get proper sleep. We are still learning much about what happens during sleep—when you slip into the subconscious and disconnect with your current reality. One can be sure that for those who have sleep apnea, with a lack of proper stages of sleep and oxygen to the brain for prolonged periods of time, brain health will be at risk. Sleep apnea may present as daytime fatigue, loud snoring that alternates with silence, irregular sleep, headaches, poor attention, and many other signs that science is still working out. Even with symptoms of obstructive sleep apnea, requesting this test of your health care team could potentially come with some push back as there may be a significant amount of insurance approval and administrative burdens in coordination of this non-invasive testing.

Systemic Inflammation

Tenth, abnormal or prolonged activation of the body's immune or inflammatory system needs to be evaluated. When it comes to abnormal inflammation in the body, there are many causes. When present, the inflammation in your body needs to be discovered and eliminated if at all possible. Such inflammation can come from medical conditions or from infection. Do the best you can to clear it up. At times one may have systemic inflammation that is identified and not easy to mitigate. A plethora of reasonably well-understood disease process may occur, and they will be treated to the best of medical science. Nevertheless, some of the systemic inflammation will persist. This category is simply not as easy to fix as the other categories, so these afflicted individuals need to pay extra attention to all the other categories.

Hypercoaguable State

Eleventh, for some of you reading this work, your genetic code may carry a defect. This defect may be as obvious as forming blood clots that go to your lungs, blood clots in the legs, multiple miscarriages, the onset of memory problems or dementia, or it can be as sinister as the first MRI of your brain showing a significant amount of damage that has already been done. Much of this damage you may have been unaware of. Before identification of this type of problem, much of this damage may have happened as daily micron strokes. Repeated damage will end up killing off functional units of your brain. Fear not! We have had clients of age sixteen and up who, after identification of this unique problem in their genetic codes, have been able to avoid micron strokes, strokes, and blood clots. Some, plagued by miscarriages, have successfully given birth to children after the attention to the details. Some clients in this category have also experienced a reversal in their memory problems after identification and treatment of this condition.

You may be in for a very challenging road if your health-care team and possibly a blood specialist are not fully aware of the extent of these very important biochemical-hematologic-phys-iological interactions in your blood system. Often, one may find a case with extensive brain/memory damage and positive hypercoaguable state, and yet the health-care team will continue with observation as no single event was profound or resulted in obvious debilitation. Simply be wary when you have a medical problem with no direct answer (memory or abnormal brain MRI) and are given a path of observation. Your observation may be a sliding slope into a facility to provide the care your damaged mind can no longer provide. The hypercoaguable state is the most exciting category, as future funding may allow us to unlock connections here to many problems that are diagnoses of exclusion.

Too often health-care providers cannot prove you have a certain disease. They simply state that they have considered possible diseases and excluded them. Because you don't have disease A, B, or C, you must have disease X. But just because your condition isn't caused by A, B, or C doesn't mean it's caused by X. Lou Gehrig's disease, motor neuron disorder (Stephen Hawking's current diagnosis), multiple sclerosis, Parkinson's disease—these are all terms that describe a variety of cerebrovascular events. These descriptive terms represent the results of strokes and micron strokes to very important functional units. We have approval and are working to publish the data of a case series involving the above diagnoses as connected, with a complete and thorough evaluation. A direct etiology for a medical condition could be of great value in treatment, as compared to a diagnosis of exclusion and observation.

Conclusion

This work is not presented as a loosely organized statement of opinion. My understanding of the problem of dementia is at times difficult to put into words. The complex interaction of multiple events and facts at the same time in a unique individual often amazes me.

Consider for a moment that the next person you meet has never seen or eaten cantaloupe. It would be difficult to describe to them what cantaloupe tastes like. You may find that something you understand and know very well is difficult to put into words. The work above is putting into words what needs to be done in the prevention of dementia.

There are so many critical details and specific goals of the unique individual that need to be addressed and then thoroughly evaluated. When you are given advice from your health-care team, ask them, "Upon what principles do you base your current decision?" You may find your visit will take a turn of attention to the accurate facts. We have covered the primary categories that need to be addressed for accurate Alzheimer's and dementia prevention; the secondary categories contain a significantly greater number of details and events. Should one complete the primary categories and still not have any success over a short period of time or there is no ability to surmise the main culprit in the brain damage, then begin investigation of the secondary categories.

Made in the USA
Columbia, SC
05 February 2021